Staying Well

New Readers Press

This book was produced in
collaboration with the
**American Institute for
Preventive Medicine.**

Copyright © 1994
New Readers Press
Publishing Division of Laubach Literacy International
Box 131, Syracuse, New York 13210-0131

Information graphics by Shane Kelley
Illustrations by Richard Ewing

9 8 7 6 5 4 3 2 1

Library of Congress Cataloging-in-Publication Data

Staying well / [American Institute for Preventive
Medicine (AIPM)].
p. cm. — (For your information)
ISBN 1-56420-027-2
1. Self-care, Health. 2. Health behavior. 3. Health.
I. American Institute for Preventive Medicine.
II. Series: For your information (Syracuse, N.Y.)
RA776.95.S73   1993
613—dc20   93-34773
                                        CIP

Contents

Preface

Information is power.

Being informed means being able to make choices. When you can make choices, you are not helpless. Having information is the first step toward being in control of a situation. It is a way to get more out of life.

The For Your Information series, also called FYI, seeks to provide useful information about a variety of topics. These topics all have something in common—they affect people's lives in major ways.

This book, *Staying Well,* discusses issues that affect everyone—health and safety. It gives useful information and suggestions for making good choices for your health.

The books in the For Your Information series are developed with experts from lead agencies in each topic area. This book was developed with help from the American Institute for Preventive Medicine (AIPM). AIPM develops and provides wellness

programs and publications. It is based in
Farmington Hills, Michigan.

Thanks to the following people for their
contribution to the content of *Staying Well:* Don
R. Powell, Ph.D., of AIPM; and Elaine Frank,
M.Ed., R.D., of AIPM.

And special thanks to Maria Collis for her
writing.

In this book

- Words in **bold** are explained in the glossary
  on pages 92–96.
- At the end of some chapters, you'll find
  resources for help or for more information.

Introduction

You can take charge of your health. Many things can harm your health. But you can avoid a lot of them. Your health problems may have something to do with your family history. But you don't have to have the same problems as your parents and grandparents.

Best of all, you can learn good health habits. This book covers eight steps to good health:

1. knowing how healthy you are
2. eating a healthy diet
3. exercising two or three times a week
4. keeping your weight down
5. not smoking

6. learning how to handle stress
7. knowing what is safe and what is not safe on the road, at home, and at work
8. seeing a doctor before you get sick

When you have good health habits, you are practicing **prevention.** Prevention is doing what you need to do to stay well.

Staying healthy is work. But it's worth it. Did you know that:

- when people die young, it's almost always because of how they lived?
- many people suffer or die from things that doctors can help?
- it's harder and it costs more to cure you than to keep you from getting sick?

Many people don't have good health habits. They don't think it matters. Do you? Do you think that:

- only other people get sick?
- people die when it's time, no matter what they do?
- doctors cost more than you can pay?
- you're afraid of doctors?
- you don't have time to go to the doctor?

If you think any of these things, you may need to pay more attention to your health. This book can help you do that.

Everything about staying well isn't known. New things are learned every day. But you can add years to your life from what is known today. This book can get you started. The rest is up to you.

Chapter 1

How Healthy Are You?

Knowing about your own health is the first step to staying well. Your doctor can help you find out how healthy you are. (For advice on how to find a doctor if you don't have one, look at Chapter 8 on page 70.)

Your doctor can help you spot the warning signs of trouble. He or she can give you shots and tests to keep you from getting sick. But you have to help your doctor and yourself. Here are some things you can do:

- take care of yourself
- watch for warning signs of bad health

- know what health risks go with your age, sex, and lifestyle
- know your family history

This book can't tell you everything about staying well. It can only give you some general ideas. You need to be aware of your own health.

This chapter is about what you need to look out for. Chapter 8 tells how to get help from a doctor.

What You Can Do

Take the self-test on page 12 to see how well you know your own health.

Look at the questions you answered "No" or "Don't know" to. You may want to read the chapters on those topics first.

This information can help your doctor, too. It will give him or her a better picture of your health needs.

When to Get Help

If you or someone in your family has any of these problems, get medical help right away:

- strange lumps or swelling
- breast lumps or pain
- **blackouts**

✔ Self-Test

Check under "Yes," "No," or "Don't know" for each
question.

	Yes	No	Don't know
Do you eat right? (see Chapter 2)	___	___	___
Do you exercise regularly? (see Chapter 3)	___	___	___
Are you overweight? (see Chapter 4)	___	___	___
Do you smoke? (see Chapter 5)	___	___	___
Is your life stressful? (see Chapter 6)	___	___	___
Is your home safe? (see Chapter 7)	___	___	___
Is your workplace safe? (see Chapter 7)	___	___	___
Have you had a **checkup** in the last three years? (see Chapter 8)	___	___	___

- dizzy spells
- blood in urine or stools (feces)
- swollen ankles
- losing or gaining weight for no reason

If these problems last more than a few days, get medical help:

- nosebleeds
- earaches
- feeling very depressed
- hoarse voice or trouble swallowing
- urinating too often, or pain when urinating
- a cold, sweating, or fever
- hoarseness or coughing
- stumbling around
- not sleeping, or feeling tired for no reason
- feeling thirsty all the time
- shaking
- pressure or pain in the chest
- having bowel movements all the time, or not being able to

You are the best judge of how you feel. Call a doctor or clinic if you think something is wrong. In an emergency, go to a hospital emergency room.

Chapter 2

Healthy Eating

Healthy eating means good **nutrition.** Nutrition is what you eat and how your body uses the food. Good nutrition is one of the best things you can do to keep in good health. Good nutrition gives you:

- the energy you need to live each day
- the strength to fight off sickness
- the material your body needs to grow and repair itself
- a healthy feel and look

You get good nutrition from a healthy diet. Your eating habits are your diet: what you eat, how much, and how often. A good diet can help lower your risk of some diseases. A bad diet can raise your risks. The following diseases have all been linked to diet:

- **high blood pressure**
- **heart disease**
- **diabetes**
- some cancers
- **osteoporosis** (a bone disease)

Your family history often plays a part in whether you will get a certain disease. But you can control or even prevent some diseases by eating well.

What Is a Healthy Diet?

The United States government has created a pyramid to show a healthy diet. It's called the **Food Guide Pyramid** (page 16). Like a pyramid, your diet is made up of building blocks. The blocks at the bottom stand for the foods you need the most of every day: breads, grains, pasta, fruits, vegetables. You should eat or drink less of what is near the top of the pyramid: meat, dairy foods, fats, sweets.

Try to:

- eat many kinds of foods
- not eat too much of one food

Food Guide Pyramid

A guide to daily food choices

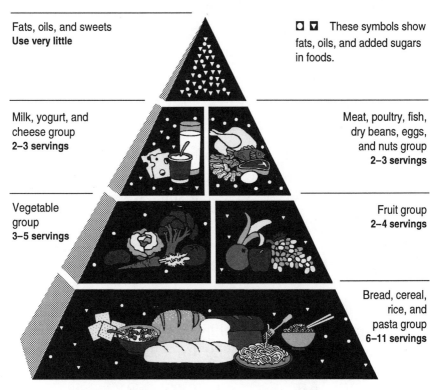

Fats, oils, and sweets
Use very little

◻ ◪ These symbols show fats, oils, and added sugars in foods.

Milk, yogurt, and cheese group
2–3 servings

Meat, poultry, fish, dry beans, eggs, and nuts group
2–3 servings

Vegetable group
3–5 servings

Fruit group
2–4 servings

Bread, cereal, rice, and pasta group
6–11 servings

The Food Guide Pyramid can help you eat a balanced diet. As you plan your meals, be sure to include items from each group. The Pyramid lists the number of servings from each group you should eat each day.

If you miss out on a certain group, you can always fill in with a snack. For example, if you've only had three fruits or vegetables, snack on an apple, or some carrot sticks.

All the food groups in the Pyramid are important. You need the least amount of fat and sugar, though.

SOURCE: U.S. Department of Agriculture/U.S. Department of Health and Human Resources

- change your eating habits slowly if you
  need to change them

A Balanced Diet

A balanced diet is a healthy diet. That
means eating the right food in the right
amounts. The Food Guide Pyramid shows the
parts of a balanced diet. Many people eat
healthy food, but they don't eat enough of some
foods. They may also eat too much of other
foods. The rest of this chapter tells you how to
eat a balanced diet.

Maybe you think you don't have time to
make healthy meals. Maybe you can't always
find good fruits and vegetables. You are not
alone. Many North Americans don't get enough
fiber, vitamins, minerals, or water. Here are
some "Whys" and "Hows" for getting what you
need.

Nutrients

Nutrients are the good things your body gets
from food. There are six basic nutrients:

1. protein
2. carbohydrates
3. vitamins

4. minerals

5. water

6. fat

Fiber is another important part of good health, but it is not a nutrient.

If you eat a balanced diet, you get all the nutrients you need.

Getting enough protein. Protein helps build and repair muscles. It also makes special blood cells (**antibodies**) that fight infection and disease. You need protein for healthy blood.

You get protein from meat, fish, cheese, eggs, other dairy products, beans, and nuts. There is some protein in grain products and vegetables.

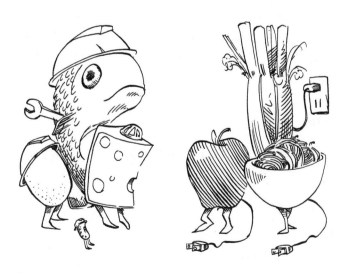

Getting enough complex carbohydrates. Complex carbohydrates are the best source of energy. They help your body work. You get complex carbohydrates from fruits, vegetables, and grain products such as whole-grain breads, cereals, rice, and pasta.

Getting enough vitamins. Every part of your body uses vitamins. You need them for healthy eyes, skin, blood, muscles, bones, and nerves. Vitamins also help your body **digest** food and fight infection.

There are 13 vitamins you should get every day. The 5 most important are:

- vitamin A
- vitamin B1 (thiamine)
- vitamin B2 (riboflavin)
- vitamin B3 (niacin)
- vitamin C

If you get enough of these 5 vitamins, you probably get the rest in the same foods. The chart on page 20 shows what foods have each vitamin. Some people also take vitamin pills or **multivitamins.**

Getting enough minerals. Your bones, teeth, and nails are made up mostly of minerals. Like vitamins, minerals help your body do its work

Vitamin	Food Source
A	liver, eggs, enriched milk and dairy products, dark green vegetables, deep yellow fruits and vegetables like apricots, peaches, cantaloupe, carrots, yams, pumpkin, squash
B1	meat (especially pork), liver, fish, green peas, beans, collard greens, oranges, asparagus, whole grains, wheat germ, nuts, yeast
B2	liver, kidneys, lean meat, chicken, tuna, sardines, milk and dairy products, eggs, dark green vegetables, whole grains, beans
B3	liver, lean meat, fish, chicken, turkey, milk, eggs, nuts, beans, dark green vegetables, whole grains
C	oranges, tangerines, grapefruit, strawberries, cantaloupe, brussels sprouts, broccoli, green peppers, collard greens, cauliflower, cabbage, tomatoes, asparagus

and digest food. Minerals also help your brain work.

There are 11 minerals you should get every day. The 2 most important are calcium and iron. If you get enough calcium and iron, you probably get the rest in the same foods.

Many vitamin pills also include minerals.

The chart on page 22 shows what foods have calcium and iron.

Getting enough water.

- Water carries nutrients to the parts of your body that need them.
- Water has minerals.
- Water helps your body digest food.
- Water carries waste out of your body.
- Water keeps your nose, mouth, throat, and other parts of your body from getting dry.
- Water helps control your body temperature. It cools your body when you sweat.

Most adults need to drink six to eight glasses of water a day. Here are some ways to enjoy drinking water more:

- Drink water with a slice of lemon or lime.
- Add fruit juice to water.
- Drink sparkling water or mineral water.
- Drink water from a glass you like.

Calcium sources	Iron sources
• milk, yogurt, cheese	• red meat
• other dairy products	• fish, shellfish
• sardines	• chicken
• salmon with the bones	• turkey liver
• clams	• kidney
• oysters	• enriched breads
• tofu	and cereals
• green leafy vegetables	• egg yolks
• broccoli	• green leafy vegetables
• kale	• dried fruits
• oranges	• blackstrap molasses
• tangerines	
• grapefruit	

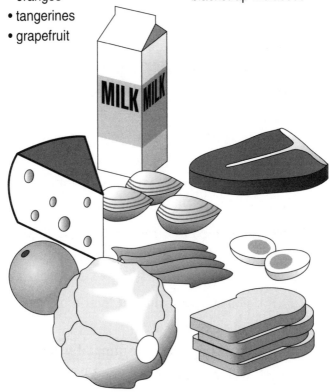

- Eat foods that have a lot of water in them. Some examples are iceberg lettuce (95% water), cantaloupe (91% water), and raw carrots (88% water). Juices, soups, and other fruits and vegetables also contain a lot of water.

Getting more fiber

- Fiber passes through your body and leaves as waste. Along the way, it helps the **digestive tract** muscles.
- Fiber fights constipation (when your body has trouble getting rid of solid waste).
- Fiber can lower your risk of **colon** cancer (cancer of the large intestine). It helps carry waste out of the large intestine.
- Fiber can lower your risk of **hemorrhoids.**
- Fiber can lower your blood **cholesterol**.
- Fiber can help you keep your weight down. High-fiber foods usually have less fat than other foods. They take longer to chew and are more filling, so you end up eating less.

To get more fiber:
- Eat whole-grain bread and rolls instead of white bread.
- Eat less meat and fat. You will have more room for fruits and vegetables.

- Eat salad or lightly cooked vegetables when you can. More vegetables mean more fiber. Vegetables with a lot of fiber include broccoli, carrots, potatoes, spinach, green beans, green peas, and tomatoes.
- Eat the skins on potatoes and fruits.
- Eat fruit instead of drinking fruit juice. Fruits with a lot of fiber include apples, bananas, oranges, pears, cantaloupe, and berry fruits.
- Put more beans and less beef in chili.
- Eat a bowl of oatmeal or bran cereal for breakfast instead of donuts or eggs.

Too Much of a Good Thing?

Many people love foods like cake, ice cream, and french fries. Foods like these often have a lot of salt, sugar, or fat.

A little salt, sugar, and fat in your diet is fine. But it's important to limit them. If you try cutting down on one thing at a time, it's easier.

Here are some "Whys" and "Hows" for lowering salt, sugar, and fat in your diet.

Cutting down on salt

Why: Salt (sodium) makes your body hold more water. This can raise your blood pressure.

High blood pressure can lead to **hypertension** and heart disease. Healthy people should keep salt down to help avoid high blood pressure. People who have high blood pressure or heart disease must cut down on salt.

How:

- Use less salt when you cook.
- Don't add salt to food after it is cooked.
- Learn to cook using other spices. You can buy some seasonings that are meant to replace salt. After a while, you may not miss the extra salt.
- Use fewer ready-made sauces. Make your own sauces. Use onion, green pepper, or lemon juice instead of salt.
- Some restaurants have special menus with "heart-smart" foods. Heart-smart foods are usually low-salt and low-fat.

Cutting down on sugar

Why: Your body burns calories from food. Calories are units of energy. Sugar gives your body empty calories. Empty calories give you quick energy, but no nutrients. Empty calories don't always make you feel full, either.

Extra calories turn into fat. That's why eating too much sugar can make you gain weight. Very overweight people are at greater risk of diabetes, heart disease, hypertension, gall bladder disease, and **stroke.** Sugar also leads to **tooth decay** or cavities.

How:

- Cut down on soft drinks, if you can. Or try drinking diet soft drinks. Diet soft drinks have fewer calories and do not lead to tooth decay.
- Have sweet snacks only once per day, if at all. (Better yet, snack on fresh fruits or vegetables.) Have a drink of water after eating sweets. Brushing your teeth after you eat is a good idea, too.
- Read food labels. Many foods have hidden sugar. Look for corn syrup, fructose, maltose, and lactose. You may be surprised how much sugar is in some foods.

Cutting down on fat

Your body is made up of cells. Many cells in your body have fat in them. Your body needs some fat. It protects organs like the heart and stomach. Fat carries vitamins to where your body needs them. And it helps prevent dry skin.

Most North Americans eat more fat than they need for good health. Experts say to keep fat down to 30 percent of your daily diet.

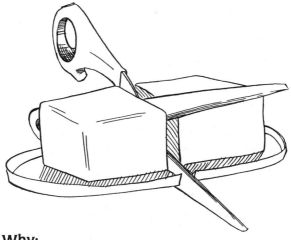

Why:

- Fat is twice as fattening as sugar. Too much fat in your diet can make you very overweight.

- Fat in your diet affects how much cholesterol is in your body. Too much cholesterol can lead to hardening of blood vessels called **arteries**. Cholesterol can also build up inside the arteries and block blood flow. That can lead to heart disease. High-fat foods have a lot of cholesterol.

- A high-fat diet raises your risk of colon cancer, breast cancer, and cancer of the uterus.

How:

- Eat less meat. Eat fish, chicken, or turkey instead of beef, lamb, or pork. Take the skin off chicken and turkey before you cook it.

- When you eat beef, choose lean cuts (pieces with less fat). Trim off fat before cooking.
- Broil or bake meat instead of frying it. Broil meat on a rack so the fat can drip off. When you are in a restaurant, choose broiled meats without heavy sauces.
- Use skim or low-fat milk instead of whole milk. Use milk instead of cream in coffee and tea.
- Use fewer eggs. Try using one egg yolk and a few egg whites in scrambled eggs and omelets. It's the yolks that have the cholesterol.
- Cut down on fried foods.
- Boil, bake, steam, or stir-fry vegetables.
- Use oil instead of shortening. Use margarine instead of butter.
- Use a non-stick pan. Use cooking spray or a little oil instead of butter, margarine, or bacon grease.
- Cut down on sour cream and mayonnaise in recipes. Try blended, low-fat cottage cheese, low-fat yogurt, or buttermilk instead.

- Cut down on oil in salad dressings. Try lemon juice or vinegar.
- Read food labels. Look for foods labeled low-fat.

Cholesterol

If you cut down on fat, you will also cut down on cholesterol. Try to avoid or limit these foods:

- meat fat, including chicken fat
- cream
- whole milk
- hard cheese
- butter
- shortening
- stick margarine
- chocolate
- coconut oil
- palm oil
- palm kernel oil

These are **saturated fats**. They are bad because they help cholesterol build up in your body.

Remember: Whatever kind of fat you eat, a little fat is all you need.

Dental Health

What you eat affects your teeth and gums. Here are some tips for healthy teeth and gums:

- Eat a balanced diet.
- Avoid sweets and regular sodas.
- Drink water or brush your teeth after eating sweets.
- See a dentist twice a year.
- Follow the dentist's advice about how to brush and floss your teeth, and how often to do it.
- Use a fluoride toothpaste to help fight cavities.
- Buy a new toothbrush every three to four months.

To find out more

Call your local agricultural (or "cooperative") extension service. The number should be in your phone book. Or contact:

Human Nutrition Information Service
Room 325-A 6506 Belcrest Road
Hyattsville, MD 20782
(301) 405-2139

American Dietetic Association
Nutrition Hotline
(800) 366-1655

Chapter 3
Exercise

Exercise is important for good health. Here's why. Exercise:

- helps make your heart and muscles strong
- is good for bones, joints, and blood flow
- helps you digest food and burn extra calories
- helps you deal with stress
- can lift your spirits and make it easier for you to handle pain
- is good for your self image—how you see yourself

Even if you eat right, don't smoke, keep your weight down, and get good health care, you still need exercise.

How Often Should You Exercise?

Regular exercise is the best exercise. That means you don't go for long without exercise. Exercising three times a week for 20 minutes is better than exercising once a week for an hour. Finding someone to exercise with may help you stick to a regular time.

What Is Good Exercise?

Good exercise makes your heart pump faster. This is called **aerobic exercise.** Aerobic exercise can be:

- walking (quickly, working hard)
- jogging
- running
- swimming
- riding a bicycle
- dancing

Many other sports can be aerobic, too. Aerobic exercise helps your heart. It can also help you lose weight. Your body burns calories faster for several hours after aerobic exercise.

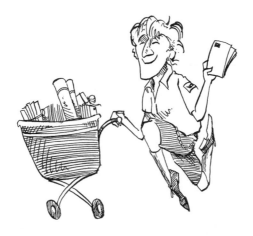

Some jobs give you good exercise. If you use your body in your work, you may get enough exercise there.

Walking

Almost anyone can walk for exercise. All you need is a good pair of shoes. Hold your head up and let your arms swing. Walk quickly, so your heart pumps faster. It's great exercise.

Aerobics

Aerobics can be a kind of dancing. Aerobic dance is good exercise. But the jumping and bouncing in high-impact aerobics can hurt your joints. Many health clubs and gyms offer low-impact aerobics.

In low-impact aerobics you:

* keep your feet close to the floor
* do little or no jumping
* use your arms more than in other kinds of aerobics

Stick to low-impact aerobics if you are over 30, overweight, or have knee problems.

Exercising at home

Many jobs around the home include some physical exercise. But you can also do aerobic exercise in your home.

Some TV ads try to sell you exercise equipment to use at home. Some of these products are good. Some aren't. Before you buy anything, ask yourself these questions:

* Will I really use it? Or will I get bored in a week or two?
* Can I afford it?
* Is the company that makes or sells the product honest? (Find out how to get your money back if you return the product.)
* Does the equipment do what it says? (Try it out.) Do you like it? Do you know anyone else who has it? Are they happy with it?

What Is Best for You?

The best exercise for you is something you like. If you like it, you'll stick with it. If you don't like exercise classes or lifting weights, you may like walking or jogging. If you are overweight, you may like swimming or water aerobics better than running. Your body weighs less in water, and you don't risk hurting your back, knees, or ankles.

Whatever exercise you choose, remember these tips:

- Talk to your doctor about what you plan to do. This is very important if you have not exercised for a long time, are overweight, or have health problems.
- Pick something you can do. Walk before you run. Bike a short way, and go a little farther each time. If you need special equipment, can you get it? If you have to go to a special place, can you get there two or three times a week?
- Exercise at the same time each day. That way, exercise is part of your schedule.
- Wait at least two hours after eating before you exercise. Wait about 25 minutes after exercising before you eat.

- Exercise two or three times a week. Get
  your heart pumping faster for at least
  15 to 20 minutes each time.
- Find someone to exercise with you.
- Take it easy. Some people think exercise
  has to hurt. That's not true. In fact, you can
  hurt your body if you exercise too hard.
  Slow down if you feel out of breath.
  Ease up if you feel discomfort. Stop if you
  feel pain.
- Don't wear too many clothes. Your clothes
  should be loose and comfortable. If you are
  outside in cold weather, wear a hat and
  many layers of clothes. As you get warm,
  take off a layer of clothes.

To find out more
Call these hotlines:
   **American Running and Fitness
   Association**
   (800) 776-ARFA
         (776-2732)
   **President's Council on Physical
   Fitness and Sports**
   (202) 272-3430

Chapter 4

Keeping Your Weight Down

Your weight affects your health. Being overweight can hurt your back and knees. Extra weight puts stress on your heart, too. When you are 20 percent overweight or more, you raise your risk of high blood pressure, diabetes, and heart disease.

Are You Overweight?

Sixty million North Americans are overweight. Are you? If your weight is keeping you from doing things you want or need to, you probably are. Check with a doctor or other health care provider if you're not sure.

Here is one quick way to tell if you have too much body fat:

Pinch your upper arm, the back of your thigh, and just above your waist. If you can pinch more than an inch of skin in any one place, you probably have too much body fat.

Tips for Losing Weight

- Set a goal. Decide how much you need to lose. If it's more than 10 pounds, break it up into smaller goals. For example, if you want to lose 50 pounds, start by trying to lose 10.
- Talk to your doctor about what you plan to do. This is very important if you are very overweight or have other health problems.
- Cut down on salt, sugar, and fat. Use the tips on pages 24–29.
- Change your eating habits slowly. Change one thing at a time.
- Exercise regularly. Exercise helps you lose weight faster and feel better. Exercise does not make you more hungry.
- Don't "crash diet." Losing weight too fast hurts your heart and other organs. It can

make you feel weak and depressed. You don't learn healthy eating habits when you crash diet. So you will probably gain the weight back again.

- Plan your meals and snacks before you shop. Then make a shopping list and stick to it. Stay away from the cookie and snack lanes of the store. Don't shop when you're hungry.
- In restaurants, skip the bread. Or eat bread without butter. Ask for water. Drink it while you wait for your food. Eat only what you want. Take home the rest.
- Weigh yourself only once a week.
- Reward yourself! Changing the way you eat is hard work. Do something you enjoy. Buy or make something new to wear. Call a friend you miss. You deserve to do something nice for yourself.

Chapter 5

Quitting Smoking

Smoking causes sickness and early death. It is the major health risk you can prevent.

The Dangers of Smoking

More than 410,000 people die in the U.S. every year from smoking. Doctors say each cigarette takes 15 minutes off your life.

The picture on page 41 shows how smoking can affect your body. It tells how smoking raises your risk of some problems.

The Risks of Smoking

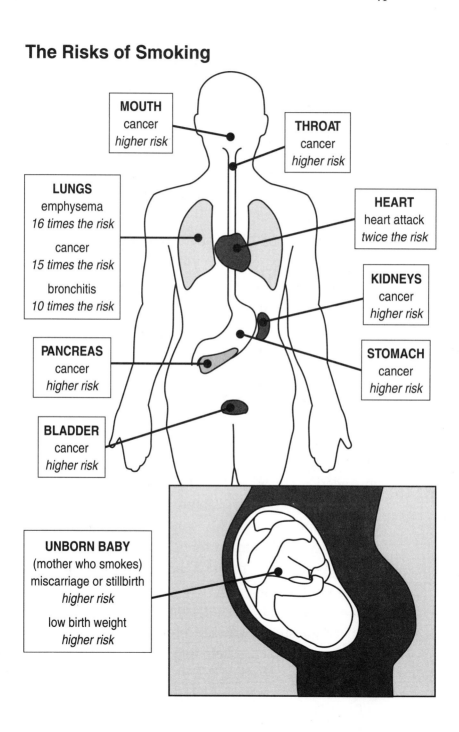

MOUTH
cancer
higher risk

THROAT
cancer
higher risk

LUNGS
emphysema
16 times the risk

cancer
15 times the risk

bronchitis
10 times the risk

HEART
heart attack
twice the risk

KIDNEYS
cancer
higher risk

PANCREAS
cancer
higher risk

STOMACH
cancer
higher risk

BLADDER
cancer
higher risk

UNBORN BABY
(mother who smokes)
miscarriage or stillbirth
higher risk

low birth weight
higher risk

Do you know that:

- cigarettes don't calm you down? **Nicotine** in cigarettes can make you jumpy. Deep breathing in and out is what calms you.
- smoking hurts people around you? People who breathe **secondhand smoke** can have the same problems as smokers. Children whose parents smoke suffer most from secondhand smoke.
- cigarettes don't help you think? Your brain gets less oxygen when you smoke. This can make it harder for you to think.
- low-tar and low-nicotine cigarettes aren't safe? Many smokers smoke more when they switch to a lighter cigarette.

How Hooked Are You?

The nicotine in cigarettes is a drug you can get **addicted** to. Once your body gets used to it, you need it. In addition, smoking is a habit. Most heavy smokers reach for a cigarette without thinking about it.

Are you addicted to nicotine? Or do you smoke more out of habit? Take the self-test on page 43 to find out.

If you checked "yes" or "sometimes" for any of these questions, you are probably addicted. You may need special help to quit.

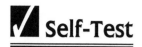 **Self-Test**

Are You Addicted?

Check under "Yes," "Sometimes," or "No" for each question.

	Yes	Some-times	No
Do you smoke your first cigarette of the day in the first half hour of the day?	___	___	___
Do you enjoy your first cigarette of the day the most?	___	___	___
Do you smoke most in the morning?	___	___	___
Is it hard for you not to smoke in "no smoking" places?	___	___	___
Do you smoke more than 16 cigarettes a day?	___	___	___
Do you smoke even when you're sick?	___	___	___
Do you inhale?	___	___	___
Do you smoke cigarettes with more than 0.5 milligrams of nicotine?	___	___	___

Quitting

Many smokers want to quit. Others don't think it's worth it. Here are some things you should know:

- Quitting won't make you gain weight. A U.S. government study showed that one-third of quitters gain weight, one-third lose weight, and one-third stay the same.
- It's never too late to quit. Your body starts to get better 12 hours after your last cigarette.

Tips for quitting

- Get rid of all cigarettes. Put away ashtrays, matches, and lighters.
- When you want a cigarette, take five slow, deep breaths.
- Drink a lot of water. Try to stay away from coffee, alcohol, and sweets. They can make you want to smoke even more.
- Get plenty of sleep and exercise. Eat healthy foods.
- Keep your mouth and hands busy. Try chewing gum or sucking on a toothpick. Eat carrots or celery sticks. Play with a paper clip or squeeze a ball.

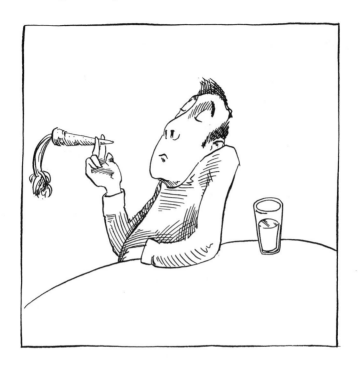

- Try a new exercise or hobby.
- Tell your family and friends you are quitting. Ask them for help if you need it.
- Feel good about quitting. Think of yourself as a nonsmoker.
- Be good to yourself. Many people "slip up." You haven't failed if you do.
- Ask your doctor about support groups for people trying to quit.

If none of these work, talk to your doctor. He or she can order medications such as nicotine patches to help you quit.

Helping someone else quit

If someone you care about is trying to quit, here's how you can help:

* Listen. Don't tell them what to do. Give advice only if they ask for it. Don't nag or yell.
* Understand that quitting isn't easy. Praise them, even if they slip up. Help them celebrate their successes along the way.
* Offer to baby-sit, cook, or do other favors during the first few days. This will take some stress off them.
* Tell them that you are proud of them.

To find out more

Call the local chapter of the American Cancer Society. You'll find the number in your phone book. For information on quitting smoking, look in the yellow pages under "Smokers." Or call:

Cancer Information Service
1-800-4-CANCER
(422-6237)

Chapter 6
Handling Stress

Do you ever feel stress? You may feel stress when something great happens, or when something bad happens. Some people feel stress in their daily lives. A little stress can help you do what you need to do. Too much can harm you. Stress can be good or bad.

Some common causes of stress are:

- having too much to do every day
- moving to a new place (home or town)
- a new job
- losing or leaving a job
- problems in relationships

- getting married or divorced
- having a baby
- the death of a loved one
- sickness or injury
- money problems
- noise

This chapter can help you understand stress. It will also help you recognize your own stress. Then you can start to deal with it.

What Stress Does to Your Body

Your body reacts to stress. You breathe faster and your blood pressure goes up. Ongoing stress can lead to aches and pains, getting sick often, and sleep problems. It can exhaust you. Two-thirds of all visits to family doctors are for problems that come from stress.

There are many physical signs of stress. Some of these are:

- tight muscles
- headaches
- stomachaches
- backaches
- **ulcers**
- tiredness
- strained eyes

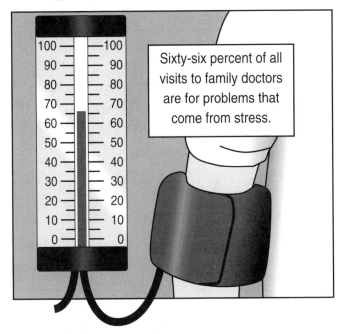

Sixty-six percent of all visits to family doctors are for problems that come from stress.

- too much sweating
- constipation or diarrhea
- fast heartbeat
- high blood pressure
- skin rashes
- urinating often
- weakness or dizziness

At its worst, stress can lead to heart disease, **colitis,** back pain, and ulcers. And stress has been linked to almost every disease that attacks the immune system. (Your immune system fights disease.) If you have any of the above symptoms, see your doctor.

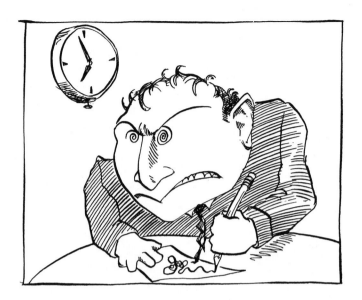

What Stress Does to Your Mind

Stress can control your life if you let it. When you feel stress, you may:

- have trouble working
- have trouble sleeping
- doubt yourself
- forget things
- have trouble concentrating
- drive carelessly
- eat more
- drink more
- smoke more
- use drugs

- feel depressed
- be irritable, anxious, or impulsive
- have mood swings
- stop caring about life

What You Can Do

You need to find ways to stop stress from taking control of your life. You can get help from a doctor or counselor. You can also do things for yourself. Here are some tips for handling stress in your everyday life:

- Talk about your feelings or problems with someone you love.
- Finish a job or chore that makes you feel good.
- Get enough sleep.
- Stay healthy—eat a balanced diet and exercise regularly.
- Take some time each day to relax. Think about a restful place, like a beach. Listen to music, stretch, take a nap.
- Look on the bright side—
  Did anything good happen today?
  Did you get anywhere on time?
  Did you get something you wanted?
  Did anyone say something nice to you?

When you feel stressed out

Do you ever feel like you're going to explode? Do you want to yell at the first person who looks at you?

Stress can get to anybody. But relaxing can help you prevent stress. Here are some tips for relaxing quickly if you start to feel stressed out:

- Count to 10. Breathe slowly and deeply for three to five minutes.
- Relax your muscles by making them tight, then letting go.
- Stretch.

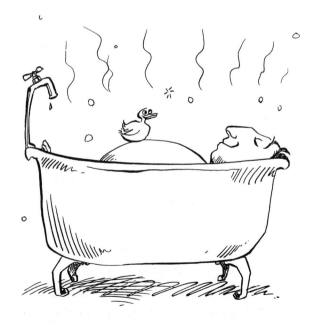

- Make a cup of herbal tea. (Herbal tea has no caffeine to make you jumpy.) Sip it slowly.
- Take a warm bath.
- Do some activity you enjoy.
- Listen to music you like.
- Take a walk.
- Play with a child or pet.

You can also learn special ways to relax, like **yoga** or **meditation.** Your library may have tapes, books, or videos about stress and relaxing.

If you worry about a lot of things, ask yourself these questions:

- What is the problem?
- Is it really a problem?
- Is it really my problem?
- How important is the problem?
- Can I do anything about it?

You may find that you can stop worrying about something by answering these questions.

Try to be a positive thinker. Remember to reward yourself for what is going right before you worry about what may be wrong. Think about the good things that will happen tomorrow. Then try to decide how you'll deal with the other things.

Managing your time

Everyone has the same 24 hours in the day. Do you feel that you need more? Knowing how to use your time well may make you feel as if you have more of it.

Here are some tips for making the most of your time:

- Plan carefully. Set goals and priorities. Keep a list of what you need to do every day. Don't put things on the list unless you really plan to do them that day. Check items off your list when you do them. That will make you feel good about getting things done.
- Try not to put things off if you can do them easily right away.
- Try to say no when people ask you to do things that might be difficult to do. Know your limits. It's OK to say no once in a while. If you have trouble saying no, remember this: You won't be able to do anything at all if you get sick.
- Plan ahead to spend time with family and friends. Try not to let other things get in the way of those plans.
- Avoid "time wasters." These may be tasks that don't really need to be done, or

spending your free time with people who don't help you relax.

Knowing When You Need Help

You can do a lot on your own to handle stress. But sometimes stress may get too bad for you to handle by yourself. That's when you need professional help. You can get help from counseling or a self-help group. Your doctor can help you find something right for you.

The first step is knowing that you need help. Here are some signs to look for:

- You feel like you have lost control of your life.
- You have problems dealing with other people.
- You feel hopeless, confused, or frustrated.
- You don't enjoy anything anymore.
- You feel great, then you feel awful (or the other way around).
- You feel depressed for weeks or months.
- You do things to hurt yourself or others.
- You have problems with sex.
- You have trouble sleeping for weeks or months.
- You feel afraid for no reason.

- You think about killing yourself.
- You think about being sick all the time.
- You drink a lot of alcohol or take drugs.

A Last Word about Stress

Everyone has stress. You may have less stress if you have a good outlook on life. Look for something to laugh about when you can. Daydream. Believe in yourself. Be a positive thinker. Positive thinkers believe things will turn out OK—or better. Since you can't usually run away from stress, learn to flow with it.

But remember that stress can be a sign of deeper problems in your life. Learn to manage your stress, but seek help to deal with the causes of your stress if you need to. Remember these important things you can do to help yourself manage stress:

- Eat a balanced diet (see Chapter 2).
- Exercise regularly (see Chapter 3).
- Sleep a regular amount each night.
- Avoid caffeine (in coffee, tea, and chocolate) and nicotine (in tobacco).
- Learn to relax.
- Learn to use your time well.
- Know when to seek help.

To find out more

- Ask your doctor for suggestions.
- Look in your local paper for support groups.
- Ask your employer if your company provides any services to help employees cope with stress.
- Look in the phone book under Social Services, Mental Health Services, or Stress Management Programs.

Chapter 7

Preventing Injury

Injury is the fourth largest cause of death in the U.S. It is the leading cause of death for people under 45. About half these people die in auto accidents. Many others die in accidents at home or at work. But you don't have to be in an accident to get hurt. Many people get injured doing everyday things.

You can make your life safer in your car, at home, and at work. This chapter has some tips to help you.

Common Causes of Accidents

1. not getting enough sleep, or waiting too long to sleep
2. being upset
3. drinking alcohol or taking certain medicines
4. working too fast
5. acting too fast or without thinking
6. using tools wrong or badly
7. not knowing how to do something
8. not paying attention
9. taking risks you don't have to take
10. very hot or very cold weather

Safety on the Road

What you can do

Safety belts. Fewer than half the people in the U.S. wear safety belts. Wear your safety belt. Make sure your child wears a safety belt. If your child is under 4 years old, put him or her in a child safety seat. Small children who are not in safety seats are 10 times more likely to die in an accident.

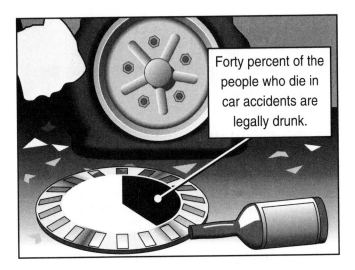

Forty percent of the
people who die in
car accidents are
legally drunk.

Drinking and driving. Forty percent of the people who die in car accidents are legally drunk. Don't drink and drive. If you drink on an empty stomach, it takes even less alcohol to make you drunk.

Motorcycles and bicycles. In states where people must wear a helmet, motorcycle deaths have gone down 30 percent. If you ride a motorcycle or bicycle, wear a helmet.

Stopping when driving. Stop often, even if you're not tired. Stop as soon as you feel tired. Pull off the road if you have to.

Other drivers. Watch out for drivers who:

- drive too fast or too slow
- start or stop suddenly

- run stop signs or traffic lights
- follow too close behind other cars
- pass other cars too fast or too slowly
- change lanes a lot or weave from left to right
- drive without lights when it is dark
- drive with their windows open in the rain or cold
- are drinking, talking, or laughing instead of watching the road

Safety at Home

In the U.S., almost 250,000 people die each year in home accidents. Here is a list of the main causes of home accidents. The causes are different for different age groups.

Age	Main cause of accidental death
0–1 year	choking or **suffocation**
1–14 years	burns or fire
14–45 years	poisoning
45–64 years	burns or fire
over 65 years	falling

Is your home safe?

Here is a safety checklist for your home. Check off the things you have already done (or do) in your home. Take steps to change things you don't check.

___ Keep a first-aid kit handy. (See page 64.)

___ Keep cleaners and other poisons in the same bottles they came in.

___ Keep things like gasoline away from stoves and heaters.

___ Keep towels, curtains, and electric cords away from stoves and heaters.

___ Don't overload electric outlets. Try to run only one cord from each outlet.

___ Don't put cords where people can trip over them.

___ Get a small fire extinguisher. Learn how to use it and keep it in the kitchen.

___ Keep ashtrays, irons, and electric curlers away from things that can catch fire.

___ Get a smoke detector if you don't have one. Put it on or near the ceiling.

___ Test the smoke detector twice a year to be sure it works. Remember to do this by doing it when you move your clocks forward and back in April and October.

___ Keep hair dryers, electric shavers, and curling irons away from water.

___ Put a nonskid mat in front of each sink.

___ Put a rubber mat or rubber stickers in the bathtub or shower.

___ Put bright lights in hallways and over stairs. If you can't do that, you can buy tape that reflects light. Put this tape on the top and bottom steps.

___ If you have a stairway, make sure it has a good handrail. If you rent in a building with a stairway, ask your landlord to put in a handrail.

___ Keep these numbers near the phone:
- police
- fire department
- poison control center
- ambulance
- clinic or family doctor

Most of these numbers are in the front of your phone book.

___ If you live in a house, test for **radon.**

Radon is a gas that can make you sick. Some homes have radon. Buy a radon test kit at the hardware store. Or call your city housing department or heating company. They can tell you more about radon and radon testing.

Your first-aid kit

You can handle many small accidents that happen at home. You need to keep some first-aid supplies on hand. Buy **generic** brands—they're usually cheaper.

What to have	Use it for
aspirin	minor aches and pains
antacid	upset stomach
baking soda	itching and sunburn
hydrogen peroxide or iodine	cuts and scrapes
adhesive bandages	cuts and scrapes
antihistamine	allergies, stuffy nose, sneezing
oral thermometer	checking body temperature
tweezers	splinters
ace bandage	sprains, twisted ankles and knees
calamine lotion	hives, insect bites, rashes
gauze bandages	large cuts, burns
cloth tape	use with gauze bandages
syrup of ipecac	poisoning (if directed to use it by a doctor or poison control clinic)

If you have children

Here are some special safety tips for homes with children.

Put these things where children can't reach them:

- cleaners and other poisons
- knives, scissors, and other sharp objects
- plastic bags
- small objects that could be swallowed

Other tips:

- Block stairways so that small children can't fall.
- Cover electric outlets with plastic covers. (You can buy covers at hardware stores.)
- Put childproof locks on drawers or cupboards where you store sharp things or cleaners. (You can buy special locks at hardware or grocery stores.)
- Put food and drinks for small children in plastic dishes.
- Don't put a child's bed or crib right under a window. The child might climb out and fall.

Lead

Your county health department can advise you about testing your home for lead. Lead in water pipes or in paint is dangerous, especially for small children.

If the pipes in your home have lead in them, run the water for a full minute before you use it. If the paint has lead in it, ask your county health department for advice.

Fire

No matter how careful you are, fire can happen. Make sure your whole family knows how to get out if there's a fire. Keep the fire department's phone number handy.

Safety at Work

If you work with heavy equipment or electricity, you know that accidents can happen. There may be other dangers in your workplace, too. Here are some tips for work safety:

- Learn how to use a tool before you use it.
- Use the right tool for the right job.
- Make sure you can see what you are doing.
- Keep your work area clean and tidy.

- Wear the right clothes for the job. Protect yourself with goggles, gloves, a hard hat, or other clothing when you need to.
- Know how and where to get help or get to safety in an emergency.

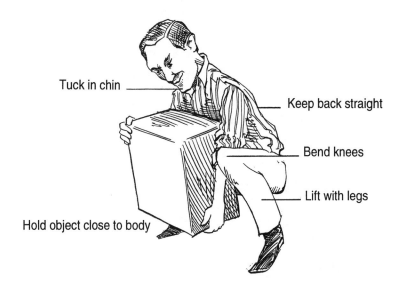

Tuck in chin

Keep back straight

Bend knees

Lift with legs

Hold object close to body

Protect your body

- Bend your knees when you lift something heavy. Hold it close to your body.
- If something is too heavy to lift, push it. Don't pull it.

- Prop one foot up on a stool or box if you have to stand for a long time.
- Don't wear high heels if you are on your feet all day.
- Put your work in front of you. Make sure it is not too high or low.
- Your lower back should rest against your chair. Try to stick your hand in behind your back just above your waist. If you can do it, you need more back support. Put a pillow or a rolled up towel behind your back.
- Your feet should reach the floor and any pedals without stretching.

Injuries without accidents

You can get hurt at work without having an accident. You can get hurt just by doing the same thing over and over. This is called **repetitive motion injury.**

Do you work on an assembly line or on a computer all day long? Do you pound a hammer or put together parts? Do you paint or use controls? If you use repeated motion in your job, here are some tips for you to remember:

- Get comfortable. Don't bend over, squat, or reach to do your job. Get a chair, table, or ladder if you need one.
- Try a different way to do things once in a while. Rest the part of you that works hardest.
- Switch hands.
- Shift your weight to the other side.
- Rest your eyes.
- Take a break if you can.
- Stretch your legs.
- Roll your shoulders.
- Stop work if you feel pain. Tell your boss or go to the health and safety office at work if there is one. Go to your family doctor if you need to.

The law and work safety

Your boss has to give you a safe place to work. That's the law. Point out safety problems. Make sure you know how to get out if there is a fire. Tell your boss if you need something to help you do your job.

Chapter 8

The Doctor's Part

When should you see a doctor? How often do you need checkups? What tests do you need? This chapter will help you answer these questions. It will also help you:

- find a doctor
- talk to your doctor
- get the most from a checkup
- know when to have tests
- know what to expect from routine tests

Finding a Doctor

It's a good idea to see the same doctor each time you go, if possible. In case you don't already have a regular doctor, here are some tips for picking one. These tips work for any kind of doctor.

- Ask friends and relatives if they know a good doctor.
- Check with the county health department or local medical society. You can find their numbers in the blue or yellow pages of your phone book. Look under headings like "Health" or "Physicians." Tell them what kind of doctor you want. You can ask for a doctor who lives near you. You can even ask for a doctor by age or sex.
- Call the doctor's office. Ask if the doctor is taking new patients. If the answer is yes, then ask these questions:
  - Does the doctor do a complete checkup on new patients?
  - How much does that first visit cost?
  - When is the office open? (Are the hours good for you?)
  - Do you pay when you see the doctor, or do you get a bill?
  - What insurance does the doctor take? (Make sure the doctor honors your insurance.)
  - Does the doctor do low-cost testing and shots?

- Is the doctor alone, or do other doctors work there, too? If the doctor is alone, does another doctor help out in an emergency?
- What hospital does the doctor use? (Can you get there?)
- How soon can you get an appointment?

You may not find the perfect doctor. But if you check on a few doctors, you will be able to make a better choice. Remember that people who work in the doctor's office are important, too. Make sure they are helpful.

You should see your doctor for routine checkups. These are checks of your health when you are not sick. A doctor who does this is a primary care physician or family doctor.

Your family doctor should know you and your **medical history.** Your medical history is your past sicknesses and injuries. It includes information about your parents, grandparents, and other family members.

Your family doctor is usually the first person you see for a health problem. You may have one family doctor, or you may go to a clinic. Either way, all your medical records should be in one place.

Most people should have a routine checkup every one or two years. Some people need checkups more often. Your doctor can tell you how often you need checkups.

Sometimes your family doctor will refer you to a **specialist** for special help. A specialist is an expert in one kind of medicine. One example of a specialist is a pediatrician. A pediatrician treats children. Another example is a cardiologist. A cardiologist treats the heart.

Having a Checkup

Good medical care starts with a checkup. Having regular checkups lets you and your doctor:

- know how healthy you are
- ask questions about your health
- find out if you have a problem
- find out if you need any special tests or exams

Parts of a checkup

1. A full medical history

   This is to find out if you or anyone in your family has ever been sick. The doctor or nurse may ask about heart problems, cancer, diabetes, and childhood illnesses. You only have to give this information

once. The doctor's office will keep it in
your file.

The doctor or nurse may also ask about
your eating and drinking habits, and if you
smoke. It's important to answer all the
questions you can.

2. Body measurements
The doctor or nurse should measure your:
- height
- weight
- temperature
- pulse (heartbeat)
- blood pressure

3. A physical exam
The doctor should check your eyes,
ears, and skin. The doctor may look at,
thump, or listen to other parts of your
body, such as your heart and lungs.

The doctor may ask you about other
parts of your body, too. He or she may ask
if you have trouble going to the bathroom.

The doctor will check out pain or other
problems. The doctor may push or poke
a spot to see if it hurts.

4. Tests
Your doctor may run some of these tests:
- a urine test (urinalysis)

- blood tests
- X rays

X rays take pictures of your bones. They can also sometimes show cancer.

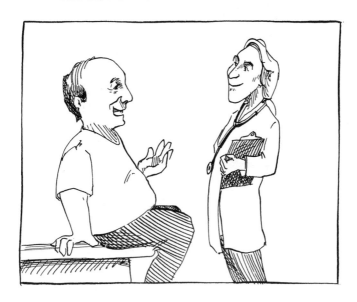

Talking with Your Doctor

After your physical exam, you and your doctor should talk about the following things.

Symptoms. Symptoms are signs that something is wrong. If you came with a problem, the doctor may ask for details about your symptoms. He or she may tell you what seems to be wrong. You may need more tests or a **prescription.**

Smoking. If you smoke, the doctor will probably tell you to quit or cut down. Ask the doctor for help in quitting if you need it.

Exercise. Exercise may be one topic. The doctor may say you need more exercise. Discuss what kind of exercise is good for you.

Diet. Your diet is another topic. If you need a special diet, make sure you understand what to eat, what not to eat, and why.

Lifestyle. Your lifestyle affects your health. The doctor may ask about your drinking habits. He or she may ask if you use drugs. If you don't want to talk to your doctor about drinking or drugs, you don't have to. But the doctor may be able to help. Or the doctor may refer you to Alcoholics Anonymous (AA) or another group.

The doctor may ask if you want testing for **sexually transmitted diseases (STDs).** There are many STDs. **AIDS** is an STD. For more information about AIDS and other STDs, see pages 88–90.

The doctor may talk to you about birth control. Tell the doctor what needs you have, if any. There are many kinds of birth control.

If you don't want to talk to your doctor about STDs or birth control, you don't have to. There are other places you can go to, such as

Planned Parenthood. Call your county health department for advice.

Tests. If you need tests, the doctor should discuss them with you. Some tests are routine. You need them even if you are healthy. Other tests look for special problems. Your doctor should explain any tests you need.

How to talk to your doctor

Your doctor is there to help you. He or she learns the most about you from what you say. It's important that you understand what the doctor says, too. Here are some tips to help you talk to your doctor:

- Tell your doctor all your symptoms. Headaches, not sleeping well, and upset stomach are examples of symptoms.
- Let the doctor do his or her job. Tell the doctor if anything has helped the problem before. Tell the doctor if anything seems to make the problem worse. But let the doctor figure out what is wrong (make the **diagnosis**).
- Don't leave anything out. Many things affect your health. Maybe you just quit smoking. Maybe your child has been sick for two weeks. Maybe you are under

special stress. Tell the doctor anything that might affect how you feel.

- Tell your doctor if you don't understand something he or she says. Ask your doctor to explain medical words or advice.

  If the doctor gives you a prescription, ask what it is for and how to take it. Ask if there are any side effects. (A side effect is something the medicine does to your body other than treat the problem.)

- Ask what to do next. How long should you take the medicine? When should you see the doctor again? Will someone call with your test results?

- Ask about things that bother you. If you can't do what the doctor tells you to do, say so. The doctor may have other ideas for you. If you worry about your weight or diet, ask what the doctor thinks.

- Call the doctor later if you have more questions.

Tests You Should Have

The chart on pages 80–81 shows tests that all men and women should have. How often you should have these tests depends on your age and medical history. Ages for each test are at the top of the charts.

Your doctor may want you to take other tests, too. Ask your doctor any questions you have. If you want advice from another doctor, get a second opinion. That means you would ask a second doctor if he or she agrees with your doctor. This is even more important if your doctor says you need an operation.

About the tests

Physical exam. This test checks your overall health. It is the first step in finding out if anything is wrong. See *Having a Checkup* on pages 73–75.

Blood pressure. The doctor or nurse wraps an empty cloth balloon (cuff) around your arm. They fill the cuff with air. The cuff gets very tight around your arm. Then they let the air out. They get a reading of your blood pressure. 140/80 is an example of a blood pressure reading. The second number should be less than 90 for good health.

Cholesterol blood test. This test shows your total blood cholesterol. The doctor or nurse takes blood from your arm with a needle. They send the blood out for testing. Your total cholesterol should be under 200.

Tests for Every Adult

Test	20–29	30–39	40–49	50+
☐ physical exam	every 3–5 years	every 3–5 years	every 2–3 years	every 2–3 years
☐ blood pressure	every 3–5 years	every year	every year	every year
☐ cholesterol blood test	every 3–5 years	every 3–5 years	every 3–5 years	every 3–5 years
☐ blood sugar test	every 3–5 years	every 2–3 years	every 2–3 years	every 2–3 years
☐ hematocrit	every 5 years	every 5 years	every 5 years	every 2 years
☐ electrocardiogram (EKG)			1 baseline	

Test	20–29	30–39	40–49	50+
☐ vision	every 3–5 years	every 3–5 years	every 2–3 years	every 2–3 years
☐ hearing	every 3–5 years	every 3–5 years	every 2–3 years	every 2–3 years
☐ urinalysis (urine test)	every 5 years	every 5 years	every 5 years	every 2 years
☐ rectal exam		every 3–5 years	every 1–2 years	every year
☐ stool blood test			every 1–2 years	every year
☐ sigmoidoscopy				every 3–5 years
☐ glaucoma screening			every 1–2 years	every 1–2 years

Blood sugar test. This test checks how much sugar is in your blood. If there is too much sugar, you may have diabetes. If there isn't enough sugar, you may have **hypoglycemia.**

There are two ways this test may be done:

- The doctor or nurse may just poke your finger and squeeze out a drop of blood, or
- You may have to eat a special diet for a few days. Then blood is taken from your arm a few times in a few hours.

Hematocrit. This test checks for **anemia** (too little iron). It counts the red cells in your blood. The doctor or nurse may just poke your finger and squeeze out a drop of blood. If they need more blood, they take it from your arm with a needle.

EKG or electrocardiogram. An EKG shows how well your heart is working. It also shows if your heart muscle is injured. This test takes just a few minutes, and doesn't hurt at all.

You take your shirt off. The doctor or nurse puts patches on your chest. The patches are attached to wires. The wires go to a machine that prints out lines. The lines show how your heart is working. This test takes between 5 and 10 minutes.

Vision and hearing tests. These tests show if your eyesight or hearing is getting worse.

Vision: The doctor may shine lights in your eyes. You may have to read letters, numbers, or pictures.

Hearing: You put on headphones. You listen to different sounds. The doctor asks about what you hear.

Urinalysis. This test checks for blood and other things in your urine. This test can show if you have tumors, infection, or diabetes.

The doctor or nurse may take a urine sample at the office. (You go in the bathroom and urinate in a cup.) Or they may ask you to bring a urine sample from home.

Rectal exam. This test doesn't usually hurt. You lie down. The doctor puts on a rubber glove and feels inside your **rectum** with his or her finger. This is to check for cancer in the colon (large intestine) and rectum. (You pass solid waste through your rectum.)

Stool blood test. You bring a stool (solid waste) sample to the doctor's office. The stool is examined to see if there is blood in it. Blood in your stool is a sign of cancer or other problems in the colon.

Sigmoidoscopy. For this test, you lie down on your side. The doctor puts a tube in your rectum. He or she looks inside. This is to check for cancer and other problems in the colon.

Glaucoma screening. Your doctor may send you to an eye doctor for this test. It doesn't hurt at all. The doctor puts drops in your eyes. Then he or she uses a machine to check the pressure. If the pressure in your eyes is too high, you may have glaucoma. Glaucoma is a serious condition that needs treatment.

Tuberculosis or TB test. This test checks for the disease **tuberculosis (TB).** The doctor or nurse pricks your arm with a needle. You watch the spot for a few days. They will tell you what to look for.

For men only

Prostate exam. The doctor feels your groin to check for tumors (lumps) in your **prostate** gland.

For women only

Breast exam by doctor or nurse. You lie down and raise your arms over your head. The doctor or nurse feels each breast and squeezes each nipple. They are checking for breast lumps.

Breast self-exam (BSE). Do this test once a month at home to check for breast lumps. Do it two or three days after your period ends. Or do it on the same day each month if you don't get a period. You can do the test in parts. But you should do it all in one day. The steps are also shown on page 87.

What to do:

1. Stand in front of a mirror. Look at your breasts. Are they the same as always? Check for dimples and scaly skin. Do your nipples leak? (It's OK for milk to leak if you are pregnant or nursing.)

2. Put your hands behind your head. Press against your head. Do you see puckers or dimples now?

3. Put your hands on your hips. Pull your shoulders and elbows forward. Bend over a little. Do you see any puckers or dimples now?

Do steps 4 and 5 in the shower.

4. Get your breasts soapy. Lift your left arm. Press the fingers of your right hand on your left breast. Begin at the outside edge. Move your fingers in small circles around

the breast. Work toward the middle of the breast. Be sure to check the whole breast. Feel under the armpit, too. Feel for any lumps under the skin. Repeat with your left hand on your right breast.

5. Squeeze each nipple. Does anything come out?

6. Now lie on your back. Put a pillow under your left shoulder. (Lying this way flattens your breast.) Repeat steps 4 and 5 lying down. Move the pillow to the right side when you check your right breast.

About breast lumps

One in 10 women gets breast cancer. But breast lumps are not always a sign of cancer. You may have **fibroid tumors** or **fibrocystic disease.** Your doctor can tell you.

Do the breast exam every month. After a while, you will be able to tell what is normal for you. Look for changes. See your doctor if you feel or see something new.

Mammogram. A **mammogram** is an X ray of your breast. It is the best test for breast cancer. A mammogram can show cancer that is too small for you to feel.

You take off your shirt and bra. You put on a hospital gown. The technician gives you a lead

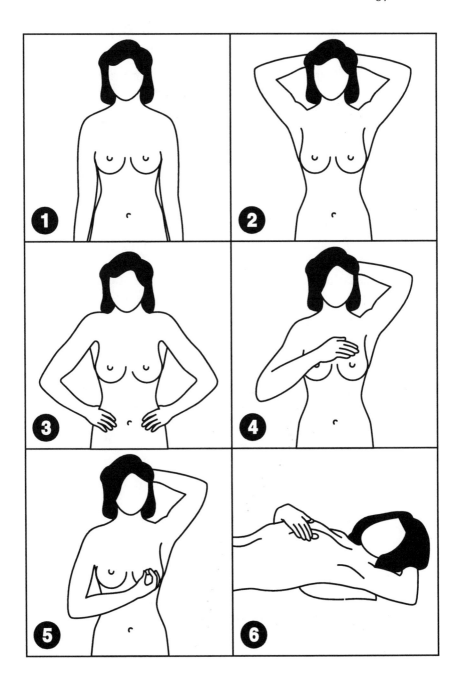

apron to protect other parts of your body. You place one breast between two flat pieces of glass. Your breast is squeezed between the pieces of glass. The X ray takes about a second. The X ray is repeated for the second breast. You may have one or two X rays for each breast.

Pap smear. A Pap smear checks for cancer in the sex organs. It helps find cancer in the vagina and **cervix.**

You lie on your back with your feet in stirrups. The doctor puts a metal tube (speculum) inside your vagina. The speculum holds your vagina open. The doctor uses a long cotton swab to scrape some cells from your cervix. The cells are tested to be sure they are normal. This test may be a little uncomfortable.

Pelvic exam. This exam checks for problems in or near your sex organs. The doctor usually does it right after the pap smear. You stay on your back with your knees up. The doctor presses on your belly and inside your vagina to feel your sex organs.

Tests for sexually transmitted diseases

You can catch a sexually transmitted disease (STD) when you have sex with someone else who has it. If you think you could have been exposed to an STD, you may want to have tests. The doctor or nurse may take a blood or urine sample.

Here are some examples of STDs:

- syphilis
- gonorrhea
- chlamydia
- genital herpes
- hepatitis B
- HIV/AIDS

About HIV/AIDS

Anyone can catch HIV. HIV is the virus (germ) that leads to AIDS. You have a higher risk of HIV/AIDS if you:

- have unprotected or unsafe sex. That is sex without using a latex condom from start to finish of the sex act.
- have had sex with many different people
- inject drugs and don't always use a brand-new needle

Your doctor can give you more information about HIV/AIDS. Or call your county health department. They can tell you more about testing for HIV.

The Centers for Disease Control National HIV/AIDS Hotline answers general questions about HIV/AIDS. They have information about prevention, testing, and treatment. They can help you find your local resources. They can also send you free materials. You can call them any day or night, any time.

English: (800) 342-AIDS
                 342-2437
Spanish (Línea Nacional de SIDA):
       (800) 344-SIDA
             344-7432
Deaf access: (800) AIDS-TTY
                      243-7889

Conclusion

Staying well isn't just luck. It takes good habits and planning ahead. Here are some points to remember:

- Eat right and get regular exercise.
- Keep your weight down.
- Don't smoke.
- Wear your safety belt.
- Look out for dangers on the road, at home, and at work.
- Know what to do in an emergency.
- Know how healthy you are.
- Get regular checkups and tests. Don't wait until you're sick to call the doctor.
- Get medical help when you need it.
- Take advice about your health only from health care professionals.
- Relax and enjoy life.

The best health care is preventive health care. That means taking care of yourself before you get sick. Remember—you can take charge of your health.

Glossary

addicted: having a strong physical need for a habit-forming drug

aerobic exercise: exercise that makes the heart pump faster and gets more air into the lungs

AIDS: Acquired Immune Deficiency Syndrome. AIDS is a breakdown of the body's immune system. It is the final stage of HIV infection and is usually fatal.

anemia: lack of iron in the blood. Anemia causes weakness and paleness.

antibodies: special proteins in blood that help the body fight infections and diseases

arteries: vessels that carry blood from the heart to other parts of the body

blackout: memory loss because of alcohol. During a blackout, a person is awake. But later, the person can't remember what happened.

cervix: the entrance to the uterus, at the top of the vagina

checkup: a visit to the doctor when a patient is not sick but wants to check their health

cholesterol: a substance in animal fat that can build up inside the body and cause heart disease

colitis: a condition in which the colon is inflamed (red, tender, swollen)

colon: part of the intestine above the rectum

diabetes: a disease that means people have too much sugar in their blood. Diabetes can cause many health problems.

diagnosis: a doctor's decision about what is wrong with a patient's body. To reach a diagnosis, a doctor may examine symptoms and run tests.

digest: turn food into substances the body can use

digestive tract: the body parts and organs that help digest food

fiber: a substance that helps the body get rid of waste and that keeps the digestive system strong

fibrocystic disease: a condition where fluids get trapped in the breasts and form cysts (pockets of fluid)

fibroid tumors: lumps of body tissue

Food Guide Pyramid: a chart that shows how much of each type of food people need to eat every day

generic: lower-cost products that have no brand name

glaucoma: an eye disease that can cause
  blindness

heart disease: weakening of the heart that can
  lead to chest pain, heart attack, or stroke. It
  is also called *cardiovascular disease.*

hemorrhoids: enlarged veins in the rectum

high blood pressure: a disease that can lead to
  heart disease and other health problems.
  It is also called *hypertension.*

hypertension: severe high blood pressure

hypoglycemia: a disease in which the blood
  sugar level drops suddenly

mammogram: an X ray of the breast to check
  for cancer

medical history: a record of all health problems
  and treatments a patient has had. It also
  includes health problems that run in the
  patient's family.

meditation: a way of focusing the mind to
  relax the mind and body

multivitamin: a pill that includes many
  different vitamins and minerals. A person
  doesn't need a prescription to get them.

nicotine: a substance in tobacco that smokers
  get addicted to

nutrients: the useful materials the body gets
  from food

nutrition: food or drink and what the body gets from it

osteoporosis: a disease that causes brittle bones

prescription: the paper a doctor gives a patient so the patient can get certain medications and drugs

prevention: what someone can do to prevent health problems

prostate: a male sex gland. It makes the fluid that is part of semen.

radon: a harmful radioactive gas. It builds up in some basements where there is not enough airflow to get rid of it.

rectum: the part of the intestine right above the anus

repetitive motion injury: injury to parts of the body that repeat the same movement over and over

saturated fat: the worst kind of fat for the body. It builds up, sometimes leading to heart disease. Saturated fats are in animal products—meat, whole milk, cheese, eggs, butter, etc.

secondhand smoke: smoke from other people's cigarettes or cigars

sexually transmitted disease, STD: any disease that is passed during sex

specialist: a doctor who is an expert in one kind of medicine

stroke: an attack during which blood doesn't flow freely to the brain. Stroke can cause brain damage, paralysis, and even death.

suffocation: not being able to breathe. This may be because something is covering the nose and mouth.

syrup of ipecac: a medicine that makes someone throw up. A person should take it only if a doctor or poison control center says to.

tooth decay: the action of certain bacteria leading to cavities. Many foods help the bacteria to multiply, but sugars are the worst.

tuberculosis, TB: a disease spread from person to person through the air. It affects the lungs and other parts of the body.

ulcers: sores either inside or outside the body. Stomach ulcers cause stomachaches and problems with digestion.

yoga: physical and mental exercise that may give you strength